Plant Based Diet Specialties

Always a New Meal With This Special Cookbook

Joanna Vinson

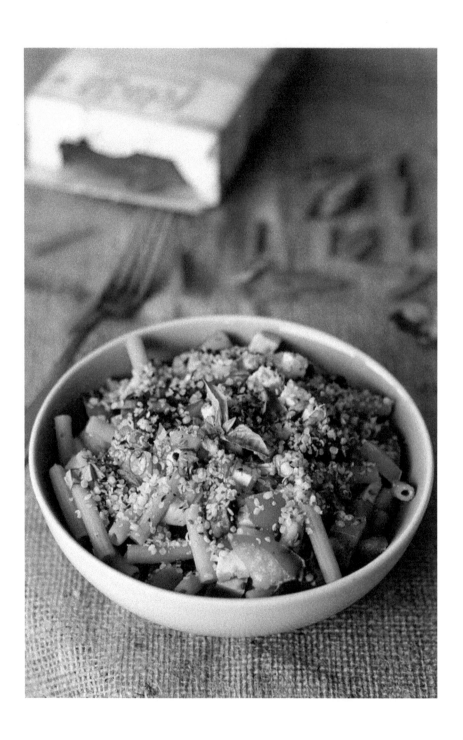

TABLE OF CONTENTS

Classic Goulash

Preparation Time: 10 minutes | Cooking Time: 15 minutes | Servings: 2

Ingredients:

- 1 cup crumbled tofu
- 2 onions, chopped
- 1 teaspoon garlic powder
- 2 cups of water
- 1 cup tomato paste
- 1cup diced tomatoes
- 1 1/2 tablespoons soy sauce
- ½ tablespoon dried basil
- 1 bay leaf
- ¼ tablespoon seasoned salt, or to taste
- 1 cup uncooked elbow macaroni

Directions:

1. Set Pressure pot to Sauté. Add crumbled tofu.
2. Add the onions and garlic powder and cook for 2 minutes.
3. Stir regularly.

4. Stir water, tomato paste, diced tomatoes, soy sauce, dried basil, bay leaf, and seasoned salt
5. into the tofu mixture.
6. Stir macaroni into the mixture, Secure the lid, and hit ―Manual‖ or ―Pressure Cook‖ High
7. Pressure for 6 minutes.
8. Quick-release when done.
9. Enjoy.

Nutrition:

Calories 425 | Total Fat 7. 5g | Saturated Fat 1. 2g | Cholesterol 0mg | Sodium 647mg | Total Carbohydrate 73. 5g | Dietary Fiber 10. 7g | Total Sugars 24. 3g | Protein 23. 8g

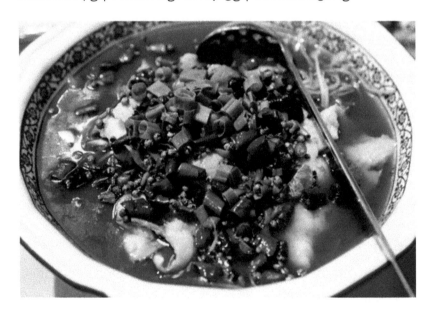

Penne with Spicy Vodka Tomato Cream Sauce

Preparation Time: 10 minutes | Cooking Time: 15 minutes | Servings: 2

Ingredients:

- ½ cup uncooked penne pasta
- 1/8 cup coconut oil
- Enough water
- 1 teaspoon garlic powder
- ¼ teaspoon paprika
- ½ cup crushed tomatoes
- ½ teaspoon salt
- 1 tablespoon vodka
- ½ cup coconut cream
- 1/8 cup chopped fresh cilantro

Directions:

1. Add penne pasta, coconut oil, water, paprika, crushed tomatoes, vodka, garlic powder, and salt to Pressure pot.
2. Place the lid on the pot and lock it into place to seal.

3. Pressure Cook on High Pressure for 4 minutes.

4. Use Quick Pressure Release.

5. Stir coconut cream into penne pasta and then stir in the fresh cilantro and combine.

Nutrition:

Calories 394 |, Total Fat 28. 7g | Saturated Fat 24. 6g | Cholesterol 23mg | Sodium 720mg | Total Carbohydrate 27g | Dietary Fiber 3. 6g | Total Sugars 5. 9g | Protein 6. 8g

Creamy Pesto Tofu

Preparation Time: 10 minutes | Cooking Time: 15 minutes | Servings: 2

Ingredients:

- ½ cup vermicelli pasta
- ¼ cup butter
- 1/2 teaspoon ground black pepper
- ¼ cup grated mozzarella cheese
- ¼ cup basil pesto
- ½ cup tofu, peeled
- Enough water

Directions:

1. Set the Pressure pot to Sauté.
2. Add butter and wait one minute to heat up.
3. Add the tofu, basil pesto sauté for one minute.
4. Stir often.
5. Add water, vermicelli pasta, and pepper.
6. Place the lid on the pot and lock it into place to seal.
7. Pressure Cook on High Pressure for 4 minutes.
8. Use Quick Pressure Release.

9. Stir mozzarella cheese.

10. Serve and enjoy.

Nutrition:

Calories 711 | Total Fat 62. 3g | Saturated Fat 52. 7g | Cholesterol 15mg | Sodium 77mg | Total Carbohydrate 32. 5g | Dietary Fiber 6. 8g | Total Sugars 8. 8g | Protein 15. 6g

Garlic Lasagna

Preparation Time: 10 minutes | Cooking Time: 20min | Servings: 2

Ingredients:

- ½ tablespoon butter
- ½ tablespoon coconut oil
- 1 small onion chopped
- 1 tablespoon garlic powder
- ½ cup ground cauliflower
- ½ cup pasta sauce
- 2 cups vegetable broth
- 1/8 cup white wine
- 1 cup of water
- 1teaspoon Italian seasoning
- 1 cup uncooked Lasagna noodles
- ½ cup shredded goat cheese divided
- 1/4 cup Parmesan cheese

Directions:

1. Set Pressure pot to Sauté.
2. Add the coconut oil and butter and allow it to sizzle.

3. Add the onions and garlic powder and cook for 2 minutes.

4. Stir regularly.

5. Add ground cauliflower and cook until about 4 - 5 minutes into Pressure pot.

6. Add pasta sauce, vegetable broth, white wine, water, and Italian seasonings.

7. Mix well.

8. Add Lasagna noodles.

9. Stir to make sure noodles are covered with the liquid.

10. Lock the lid and make sure the vent is closed.

11. Set Pressure pot to Manual or Pressure Cook on high pressure for 10 minutes.

12. When cooking time ends, release pressure and wait for steam to completely stop before opening the lid.

13. Stir in goat cheese and Parmesan cheese, but reserve about 1/8 cup Parmesan cheese if you would like to sprinkle a bit on top of the Lasagna when you serve it.

Nutrition:

Calories 325 | Total Fat 13. 4g | Saturated Fat 7. 5g | Cholesterol 31mg | Sodium 1117mg | Total Carbohydrate 34. 5g | Dietary Fiber 3. 4g | Total Sugars 9. 7g | Protein 14g

Tomato Sauce with Pumpkin

Preparation Time: 10 minutes | Cooking Time: 15 minutes | Servings: 2

Ingredients:

- ½ cup avocado oil
- 1 small onion diced
- 1 teaspoon garlic minced
- 1 cup pumpkin
- 1/8 cup fresh coriander washed and chopped
- 1 cup crushed tomatoes
- 1 tablespoon tomato paste
- ½ tablespoon dried basil
- 1/2 teaspoon salt and pepper

Directions:

1. Set the Pressure pot to Sauté.
2. Add avocado oil and wait one minute to heat up.
3. Add the onion and garlic, sauté for one minute.
4. Stir often.
5. Add the pumpkin, coriander, and sauté for one minute.
6. Stir often.

7. Add the crushed tomatoes, tomato paste, dried basil, salt, and pepper.

8. Stir well.

9. Cover the Pressure pot and lock it in.

10. Set the Manual or Pressure Cook timer for 10 minutes.

11. Make sure the timer is set to―Sealing‖.

12. Once the timer reaches zero, quickly release the pressure.

13. Enjoy!

Nutrition:

Calories191 | Total Fat 7. 6g | Saturated Fat 1. 7g | Cholesterol 0mg | Sodium 840mg | Total Carbohydrate 28. 9g | Dietary Fiber 11. 4g | Total Sugars | Protein 6g

Eggplant Fettuccine Pasta

Preparation Time: 05 minutes | Cooking Time: 25 minutes | Servings: 2

Ingredients:

- 1 tablespoon coconut oil
- 1 onion finely diced
- 1 medium zucchini chopped
- 2 cloves garlic minced
- 1 tablespoon tomato paste
- 1/2 cup vegetable broth
- 1 teaspoon dried thyme
- 1 teaspoon dried oregano
- 1 teaspoon kosher salt
- ¼ teaspoon pepper
- ½ cup diced tomatoes
- 1 cup eggplant, diced
- 1 tablespoon corn-starch
- 1 cup juice
- Shredded goat cheese for garnish

Directions:

1. Add coconut oil to the Pressure pot.
2. Using the display panel select the Sauté function.

3. When oil gets hot, add onion to the Pressure pot and sauté for 3 minutes.
4. Add zucchini and cook for 3 minutes more.
5. Add garlic and tomato paste and cook for 1-2 minutes more.
6. Add vegetable broth and seasonings to the Pressure pot and deglaze by using a wooden spoon to scrape the brown bits from the bottom of the pot.
7. Add tomatoes to the Pressure pot and stir.
8. Add eggplant to the Pressure pot, turning once to coat.
9. Turn the Pressure pot off by selecting Cancel, then secure the lid, making sure the vent is closed.
10. Using the display panel select the Manual or Pressure Cook function.
11. Use the + /- keys and program the Pressure pot for 20 minutes.
12. When the time is up, let the pressure naturally release for 15 minutes, then quickly release the remaining pressure.
13. In a small bowl, mix 1/4 cup of Pressure pot juices and corn-starch.
14. Stir into the pot until thickened.
15. Serve hot topped with shredded cheese.

Nutrition:
Calories 405 | Total Fat 14. 2g | Saturated Fat 9. 8g | Cholesterol 62mg | Sodium 1443mg | Total Carbohydrate 56. 1g | Dietary Fiber 5. 2g |, Total Sugars 8g | Protein 16. 1g

Pasta Puttanesca

Preparation Time: 05 minutes | Cooking Time: 25 minutes | Servings: 2

Ingredients:

- 1 teaspoon garlic powder
- ½ cup pasta sauce
- 2 cups of water
- 2 cups dried rigatoni
- 1/8 teaspoon crushed red pepper flakes
- 1/2 cup pitted Kalamata olives sliced
- ½ teaspoon fine sea salt
- 1/4 teaspoon ground black pepper
- 1 teaspoon grated lemon zest
- ½ cup broccoli

Directions:

1. Combine all of the ingredients in the inner cooking pot and stir to coat the pasta.
2. Lock the lid into place and turn the valve to −Sealing.
3. Select Manual or Pressure Cook and adjust the pressure to High.

4. Set the time for 5 minutes.

5. When cooking ends, carefully turn the valve to −Venting‖ to quickly release the pressure. Unlock and remove the lid.

6. Serve hot.

Nutrition:

Calories 383 | Total Fat 4. 2g | Saturated Fat 0. 9g | Cholesterol 1mg | Sodium 1269mg | Total Carbohydrate 73. 8g | Dietary Fiber 5g | Total Sugars 9g | Protein 12. 4g

Basil-Coconut Peas and Broccoli

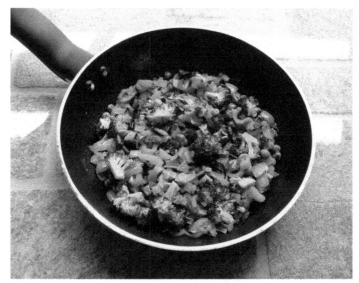

Preparation Time: 05 minutes | Cooking Time: 25 minutes | Servings: 2

Ingredients:

- 1 cup of coconut milk
- 1cup basil
- 1 bell pepper seeded and cut into chunks
- 1 leek green part only, cut into chunks
- 1 teaspoon garlic powder
- ¼ teaspoon salt
- ½ cup of water
- 1 cup noodles
- 1 cup green peas

- ½ cup broccoli florets

Directions:

1. In a blender add the coconut milk, basil, bell pepper, leek, garlic powder, and salt. Blend until smooth.
2. Pour the sauce into the inner pot and add the water.
3. Select Sauté and adjust to High heat.
4. just to a simmer, then turn the Pressure pot off.
5. Break up the noodles into 3 or 4 pieces and place them in the pot in a single layer as much as possible.
6. Layer the broccoli over the noodles.
7. Lock the lid into place.
8. Select Pressure Cook or Manual, and adjust the pressure to Low and the time to 25 minutes.
9. After cooking, quickly release the pressure.
10. Unlock the lid.
11. Gently stir the mixture until the broccoli and peas are coated with sauce.
12. Ladle into bowls and serve immediately.

Nutrition:

Calories 499 | Total Fat 31g | Saturated Fat 25. 8g | Cholesterol 23mg | Sodium 337mg | Total Carbohydrate 49. 2g | Dietary Fiber 10g | Total Sugars 12. 4g | Protein 12. 8g

Spaghetti Squash with Mushroom Sauce Pasta

Preparation Time: 05 minutes | Cooking Time: 25 minutes | Servings: 2

Ingredients:

- ½ tablespoon avocado oil
- 1 cup mushrooms
- 1 cloves garlic minced
- 1/8 cup finely chopped onion
- ¼ cup crushed tomatoes
- 1 teaspoon Italian seasoning blend
- 1 teaspoon garlic powder
- ½ teaspoon dried basil
- ½ teaspoon of sea salt
- ½ teaspoon ground black pepper
- 1/4 cup vegetable broth
- 1 bay leaf
- 1 cup spaghetti squash washed and dried
- 1 tablespoon tomato paste
- 1 tablespoon grated Parmesan cheese
- 1 tablespoon fresh parsley

Directions:

1. Select Sauté (Normal), once the pot is hot, add the avocado oil, mushrooms, garlic, and onions.
2. Sauté, stirring continuously, for about 5 minutes or until the mushrooms are browned.
3. Add the crushed tomatoes, Italian seasoning, garlic powder, basil, sea salt, black pepper, and vegetable broth to the pot.
4. Using a wooden spoon, stir and scrape the bottom of the pot to loosen any browned bits.
5. Add the bay leaf.
6. Using a paring knife, pierce the spaghetti squash 4 or 5 times on each side to create holes for venting the steam.
7. Place the squash in the pot and on top of the sauce.
8. Cover, lock the lid and flip the steam release handle to the sealing position.
9. Select Manual or Pressure Cook (High) and set the cooking time to 8 minutes.
10. When the cooking time is complete, allow the pressure to release naturally for 20 minutes and then quickly release the remaining pressure.
11. Open the lid.
12. Using a slotted spoon, carefully transfer the squash to a cutting board and set aside to cool.
13. Add the tomato paste to the pot and stir.

14. Select Sauté (Less or Low), replace the lid, and let the sauce simmer for 6 minutes.
15. While the sauce is simmering, slice the cooled squash in half and use a spoon to scoop out the seeds.
16. Using a fork, scrape the flesh to create the noodles.
17. Transfer the noodles to a colander to drain, pressing down on the noodles with paper towels to expel any excess moisture.
18. Transfer the noodles to a serving platter.
19. Remove and discard the bay leaf.
20. Ladle the sauce over top of the noodles and garnish with the Parmesan and parsley.
21. Serve warm.

Nutrition:

Calories 115 | Total Fat 4. 1g | Saturated Fat 2. 2g | Cholesterol 10mg | Sodium 893mg | Total Carbohydrate 13. 9 | Dietary Fiber 3. 6g 13% |Total Sugars 6. 1g | Protein 8. 5g

Smoked Tofu and Cherry Tomatoes

Preparation Time: 05 minutes | Cooking Time: 25 minutes | Servings: 2

Ingredients:

- 1 tablespoon coconut oil
- 1 small onion finely diced
- 1/2 cup dry red wine
- 3 cups vegetable broth
- 1 1/4 cups coconut cream
- 1 /2 teaspoon salt
- 1 tablespoon fresh dill
- 1 cup fettuccine pasta, broken in half
- 1 cup cherry or grape tomatoes halved
- 2 cups smoked tofu sliced and cut into bite-sized pieces
- Freshly ground pepper

Directions:

1. Add coconut oil to the Pressure pot.
2. Using the display panel select the Sauté function.
3. Add onion and red wine to the pot and deglaze by using a wooden spoon to scrape any brown

4. bits from the bottom of the pot.

5. Add vegetable broth, coconut cream, salt, and herbs to the pot and stir to combine.

6. Carefully fan the pasta in the pot and ensure it is completely submerged.

7. Add the halved cherry tomatoes in a single layer, do not stir.

8. Turn the pot off by selecting Cancel, then secure the lid, making sure the vent is closed.

9. Using the display panel select the Manual or Pressure Cook function.

10. Use the + /- keys and program the Pressure pot for 5 minutes.

11. When the time is up, let the pressure naturally release for 5 minutes, then quickly release the remaining pressure.

12. Gently stir the pasta, breaking up any clumps.

13. Fold in smoked tofu pieces and serve immediately garnished with freshly ground pepper and additional herbs.

Nutrition:

Calories 501 | Total Fat 31g | Saturated Fat 25. 6g | Cholesterol 31mg | Sodium 1182mg | Total Carbohydrate 40g | Dietary Fiber 3. 7g | Total Sugars 9. 7g | Protein 13g

Cheesy Creamy Farfalle

Preparation Time: 05 minutes | Cooking Time: 25 minutes | Servings: 2

Ingredients:

- 1 cup vegetable broth
- ¼ cup coconut cream
- 1 teaspoon garlic powder
- ½ teaspoon salt
- ¼ teaspoon pepper
- 1 cup dried Farfalle pasta
- 1 cup pasta sauce
- ¼ cup goat cheese shredded
- 1 cup mozzarella cheese shredded
- ½ cups fresh kale finely chopped

Directions:

1. Layer vegetable broth, coconut cream, garlic powder, salt, pepper, and Farfalle pasta in that order in the pot-- do not stir.
2. Ensure all pasta is submerged.
3. Secure the lid, making sure the vent is closed.

4. Using the display panel select the Manual or Pressure Cook function.

5. Use the + /- keys and program the Pressure pot for 6 minutes.

6. When the time is up, let the pressure naturally release for 6 minutes, then quickly release the remaining pressure.

7. Stir in the pasta sauce and kale.

8. Add the cheeses, 1/3 cup at a time, stirring until fully melted and incorporated.

9. Serve hot garnished with finely chopped kale

Nutrition:

Calories 365 | Total Fat 15g | Saturated Fat 9. 4g | Cholesterol 12mg | Sodium 1586mg | Total Carbohydrate 44. 3g | Dietary Fiber 5. 4g | Total Sugars 14. 3g | Protein 13. 8g

Basil Pesto Mushrooms Pasta

Preparation Time: 10 minutes | Cooking Time: 22 minutes | Servings: 2

Ingredients:

- 1 tablespoon coconut oil
- ½ teaspoon garlic powder
- ½ cup mushrooms
- ½ cup cherry tomatoes
- 1 cup pasta
- ½ cup basil pesto
- 1/8 bunch fresh mint
- Salt and pepper to taste
- Enough water

Directions:

1. Set Pressure pot to Sauté.
2. Add coconut oil when it gets hot then add garlic powder.
3. Stir regularly.
4. Add mushrooms and cook until about 4 - 5 minutes, cherry tomatoes, basil pesto, fresh mint, salt, and pepper.
5. Add water and pasta.

6. Lock the lid and make sure the vent is closed.

7. Set Pressure pot to Manual or Pressure Cook on High Pressure for 15 minutes.

8. When cooking time ends, release pressure and wait for steam to completely stop before opening the lid.

Nutrition:

Calories 259 | Total Fat 8. 5g | Saturated Fat 6. 1g | Cholesterol 47mg | Sodium 21mg | Total Carbohydrate 38. 1g | Dietary Fiber 1g | Total Sugars 1. 7g | Protein 8. 5g

Pressure pot Spaghetti

Preparation Time: 20 minutes | Cooking Time: 15 minutes |
Servings: 2

Ingredients:

- 1 tablespoon coconut oil
- ½ cup tofu
- ½ onion, diced
- ½ teaspoon garlic powder
- ¼ teaspoon dried thyme
- ¼ teaspoon dried basil
- ¼ teaspoon salt
- Freshly ground black pepper
- ½ cup jarred spaghetti sauce
- 2 tablespoons tomato paste
- 1 cups vegetable broth
- 2 tablespoon goat cheese, plus extra for serving
- 6 ounces of spaghetti noodles

Directions:

1. Press Sauté on your Pressure pot.
2. Add the coconut oil and tofu to the Pressure pot.
3. Cook for about 3 minutes, stirring and breaking up with a spoon occasionally.

4. Add the chopped onion.

5. Stir, and cook for about 4 minutes.

6. Stir in the garlic powder, thyme, basil, salt, pepper, spaghetti sauce, tomato paste, broth, and goat cheese.

7. Stir very well.

8. Turn off the Pressure pot.

9. Break the noodles in half, and layer them in the tomato mixture, ensuring they are covered by the liquid.

10. Press Pressure Cook and set the timer for 8 minutes.

11. Place the lid on the Pressure pot, and turn the valve to Sealing.

12. When the timer goes off, very carefully do a forced pressure release, cover your hand with a kitchen towel, and gently release the steam.

13. When you hear the float valve drop down, all of the pressure is released.

14. Open the lid to the Pressure pot.

15. It may look like there is a bit too much liquid, but just stir until it all comes together.

16. If it's still too much liquid for you, press Sauté and cook to reduce for 2 minutes.

17. Divide into bowls, and serve topped with more goat cheese.

Nutrition:

Calories 522 | Total Fat 22. 3g | Saturated Fat 13. 9g | Cholesterol 92mg | Sodium 817mg | Total Carbohydrate 54. 9g | Dietary Fiber 2g 7% | Total Sugars 4. 6g | Protein 27g

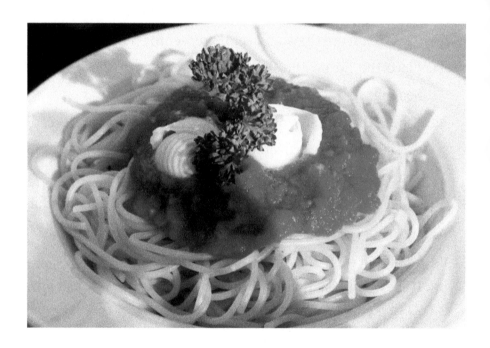

Mushrooms Creamed Noodles

Preparation Time: 5 minutes | Cooking Time: 20 minutes | Servings: 2

Ingredients:

- ½ cup heavy cream
- 2 cups vegetable broth
- ½ teaspoon dried oregano
- ½ teaspoon garlic minced
- ½ teaspoon red pepper flakes
- 1 cup noodles
- 1 cup mushrooms

Directions:

1. Put ¼ cup of the heavy cream in an Pressure pot.
2. Stir in the broth, oregano, garlic, and red pepper flakes until smooth.
3. Stir in the noodles, then set the block of mushrooms right on top.
4. Lock the lid onto the Pressure pot.
5. Press Pressure Cook on Max Pressure for 3 minutes with the Keep Warm setting off.

6. When the Pressure pot has finished cooking, turn it off and let its pressure return to normal naturally for 1 minute.
7. Then use the Quick-release method to get rid of any residual pressure in the pot.
8. Unlatch the lid and open the cooker.
9. Stir in the remaining 1/4 cup heavy cream.
10. Set the lid askew over the pot and let sit for a couple of minutes so the noodles continue to absorb some of the liquid.
11. Serve hot.

Nutrition:

Calories182 | Total Fat 5. 3g | Saturated Fat 1. 6g | Cholesterol 31mg | Sodium 850mg | Total Carbohydrate 23. 9g | Dietary Fiber 1. 9g | Total Sugars 2g | Protein 10. 2g

Singapore Noodles with Garlic

Preparation Time: 15 minutes | Cooking Time: 20 minutes | Servings: 2

Ingredients:

- 1 cup vermicelli noodles
- ¼ tablespoon hot curry powder
- ½ teaspoon garlic powder
- ½ teaspoon ginger powder
- 1 tablespoon olive oil
- ½ bunch spinach
- 1 medium carrot
- ½ cup green cabbage
- ½ green onions
- 1/8 cup soy sauce
- 1 teaspoon sesame oil
- 1 teaspoon chili garlic sauce, optional

Directions:

1. Place the dry vermicelli noodles in a bowl and cover with room temperature water.
2. Let it soak for 15 minutes.

3. Drain in a colander after they have soaked and are softened.

4. Return the noodles to the bowl, cut the noodles into pieces (approximately 6 inches in length) to facilitate stir-frying later.

5. Sprinkle the noodles with curry powder and toss to coat.

6. Set noodles aside.

7. In the Pressure pot inner pot, place the heated olive oil. add the garlic powder and ginger powder.

8. Stir fry very briefly (1 minute or less) then add all of the vegetables.

9. Stir fry the vegetables until they just begin to soften.

10. Add sesame oil, water noodles, soy sauce, salt, pepper, and chili garlic sauce.

11. Lock the lid and make sure the vent is closed.

12. Set Pressure pot to Manual or Pressure Cook on High Pressure for 15 minutes.

13. When cooking time ends, release pressure and wait for steam to completely stop before opening the lid.

14. Serve.

Nutrition:

Calories 244 | Total Fat 11. 5g | Saturated Fat 1. 7g | Cholesterol 23mg | Sodium 1036mg | Total Carbohydrate 30. 2g | Dietary Fiber 4. 8g | Total Sugars 3. 3g | Protein 7. 9g

Garlic Noodles

Preparation Time: 10 minutes | Cooking Time: 15 minutes | Servings: 2

Ingredients:

- ½ cup spaghetti
- 1 cup of coconut milk
- 1 tablespoon goat cheese
- 2 tablespoon butter
- 1 teaspoon soy sauce
- 1 tablespoon honey
- 1 tablespoon oyster sauce
- 1 teaspoon olive oil
- Enough water
- Salt to taste

Directions:

1. Add the oyster sauce, honey, soy sauce, and olive oil to a bowl and stir until combined.
2. Add spaghetti, water, and salt to Pressure pot.
3. Place the lid on the pot and lock it into place to seal.
4. Pressure Cook on High Pressure for 4 minutes.

5. Use Quick Pressure Release.
6. Stir milk into Spaghetti and then stir in the cheeses until melted and combined.
7. Add sauce mix well.

Nutrition:

Calories 239 | Total Fat 11. 2g | Saturated Fat 6. 1g | Cholesterol 58mg | Sodium 199mg | Total Carbohydrate 29. 5g | Dietary Fiber 0. 1g | Total Sugars 3. 6g | Protein 5. 6g

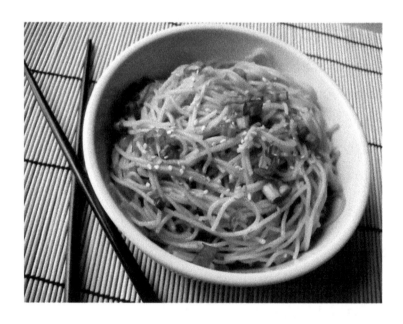

Green Goddess Pasta

Preparation Time: 10 minutes | Cooking Time: 15 minutes | Servings: 2

Ingredients:

- 1 tablespoon butter
- 1 cup mushrooms, sliced
- ½ tablespoon garlic powder
- 1 cup pasta vegetable
- 2 cups vegetable broth
- ½ cup baby kale
- ½ cup peas
- ½ cup coconut cream, cubed
- ¼ cup pesto sauce
- ¼ cup grated goat cheese

Directions:

1. Add butter to the Pressure pot, hit —Sauté‖ and once the butter is melted and sizzled, add in the mushrooms and cook for 2-3 minutes until they begin lightly brown.
2. Then, add the garlic powder and stir for another 2 minutes.

3. Next, add in the pasta vegetable and broth.

4. Top off with the kale and secure the lid and hit ─Keep Warm/Cancel‖ and then hit ─Manual‖ or ─Pressure Cook‖ High Pressure for 6 minutes.

5. Quick-release when done.

6. Stir in the peas.

7. Then, add in the coconut cream and pesto, and goat cheese and stir for about 2 minutes more until the cheese is completely melted into the sauce.

8. to a serving dish and top with grated goat cheese.

9. Enjoy!

Nutrition:

Calories 677 | Total Fat 43. 4g | Saturated Fat 20. 4g | Cholesterol 137mg | Sodium 1203mg | Total Carbohydrate 48. 6g | Dietary Fiber 3. 2g | Total Sugars 6. 1g | Protein 24. 4g

Simply Kale Lasagna

Preparation Time: 15 minutes | Cooking Time: 45 minutes | Servings: 2

Ingredients:

- 1 cup pasta sauce
- 1/8 cup water
- 1 large egg
- 2-1/2 cups shredded Italian cheese blend divided
- 1 cup ricotta cheese
- ½ cup kale
- 1 cup oven-ready (no-boil) lasagna noodles

Directions:

1. Add 1/2 cup sauce into a pan.
2. Transfer the remaining sauce to a bowl and stir in water.
3. In a large bowl, whisk the egg.
4. Stir in 1-3/4 cups Italian cheese and ricotta blend them.
5. Layer one-quarter of the noodles on top of the sauce in the pan, breaking noodles as needed to evenly cover the sauce.

6. Top with one-third of the cheese mixture with kale, then one quarter of the sauce.

7. Continue with two more layers each of noodles, cheese mixture, and sauce, gently pressing down on the noodles between each layer.

8. Finish with a layer of noodles and a layer of sauce.

9. Add 1 1/2 cups water and the steam rack to the Pressure pot. Place the baking pan on the rack.

10. Close and lock the lid and turn the steam release handle to Sealing.

11. Set your Pressure pot to Pressure Cook on High for 14 minutes.

12. When the cooking time is done, press Cancel and turn the steam release handle to Venting.

13. When the float valve drops down, remove the lid.

14. Sprinkle with the remaining Italian cheese blend.

15. Close and lock the lid and let it stand for 10 minutes or until the cheese is melted.

16. Using the handles of the rack, carefully remove the rack and pan.

17. Let Lasagna stand for 10 minutes.

18. Cut into wedges.

Nutrition:

Calories 491 | Total Fat 22. 4g | Saturated Fat 11. 3g | Cholesterol 156mg | Sodium 898mg | Total Carbohydrate 43. 8g | Dietary Fiber 4. 3g | Total Sugars 12. 1g | Protein 29. 5g

Mozzarella Lemon Pasta

Preparation Time: 05 minutes | Cooking Time: 45 minutes | Servings: 2

Ingredients:

- ½ tablespoon olive oil
- ½ teaspoon garlic powder
- 2 cups vegetable broth
- Zest of one lemon
- 1 tablespoon lemon juice divided
- 1 cup ziti noodles
- ½ cup grated/shredded mozzarella cheese
- ½ cup coconut cream
- Salt and pepper to taste
- ½ tablespoon cornstarch
- 1 tablespoon cold water
- 1 tablespoon finely chopped parsley for serving
- Additional mozzarella for serving

Directions:

1. Add olive oil to the Pressure pot.
2. Using the display panel select the Sauté function.

3. Add garlic powder, vegetable broth, lemon zest, and lemon juice to the pot and deglaze by using a wooden spoon to scrape any brown bits from the bottom of the pot.

4. Break noodles in half and fan across the bottom of the pot, making sure all noodles are submerged.

5. Turn the pot off by selecting Cancel, then secure the lid, making sure the vent is closed.

6. Using the display panel select the Manual or Pressure Cook function.

7. Use the + /- keys and program the Pressure pot for 3 minutes.

8. When the time is up, let the pressure naturally release for 10 minutes, then quickly release the remaining pressure.

9. Stir, breaking up any pasta clumps, and allow to cool slightly.

10. Add mozzarella cheese, coconut cream, and remaining lemon juice.

11. Add salt and pepper to taste.

12. In a small bowl, mix cornstarch and cold water. Stir into the pot until thickened, returning to Sauté mode as needed.

13. Serve warm topped finely chopped parsley and additional mozzarella.

Nutrition:

Calories 331 | Total Fat 21g | Saturated Fat 14. 4g | Cholesterol 4mg | Sodium 895mg | Total Carbohydrate 26. 3g | Dietary Fiber 2. 5g | Total Sugars 4g | Protein 12g

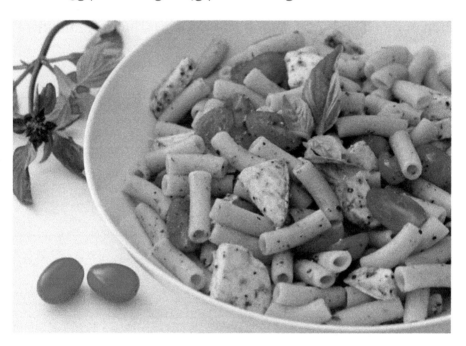

Grilled Tempeh with Green Beans

Preparation Time: 15-30 minutes | Cooking Time: 15 minutes | Servings: 4

Ingredients:

- 1 tbsp plant butter, melted
- 1 lb tempeh, sliced into 4 pieces
- 1 lb green beans, trimmed
- Salt and black pepper to taste
- 2 sprigs thyme
- 2 tbsp olive oil
- 1 tbsp pure corn syrup
- 1 lemon, juiced

Directions:

1. Preheat a grill pan over medium heat and brush with the plant butter.
2. Season the tempeh and green beans with salt, black pepper, and place the thyme in the pan.

3. Grill the tempeh and green beans on both sides until golden brown and tender, 10 minutes.
4. Transfer to serving plates.
5. In a small bowl, whisk the olive oil, corn syrup, lemon juice, and drizzle all over the food.
6. Serve warm.

Nutrition:

• Calories 352 | Fats 22. 5g | Carbs 21. 8g | Protein 22. 6g

Creamy Fettuccine with Peas

Preparation Time: 15-30 minutes | Cooking Time: 25 minutes |
Servings: 4

Ingredients:

- 16 oz whole-wheat fettuccine
- Salt and black pepper to taste
- ¾ cup flax milk
- ½ cup cashew butter, room temperature
- 1 tbsp olive oil
- 2 garlic cloves, minced
- 1 ½ cups frozen peas
- ½ cup chopped fresh basil

Directions:

1. Add the fettuccine and 10 cups of water to a large pot, and cook over medium heat until al dente, 10 minutes.
2. Drain the pasta through a colander and set aside. In a bowl, whisk the flax milk, cashew butter, and salt until smooth. Set aside.
3. Heat the olive oil in a large skillet and sauté the garlic until fragrant, 30 seconds. Mix in the peas, fettuccine,

and basil. Toss well until the pasta is well-coated in the sauce and season with some black pepper.

4. Dish the food and serve warm.

Nutrition:

• Calories 654 | Fats 23. 7g | Carbs 101. 9g | Protein 18. 2g

Buckwheat Cabbage Rolls

Preparation Time: 15-30 minutes | Cooking Time: 30 minutes |
Servings: 4

Ingredients:

- 2 tbsp plant butter
- 2 cups extra-firm tofu, pressed and crumbled
- ½ medium sweet onion, finely chopped
- 2 garlic cloves, minced
- Salt and black pepper to taste
- 1 cup buckwheat groats
- 1 ¾ cups vegetable stock
- 1 bay leaf
- 2 tbsp chopped fresh cilantro + more for garnishing
- 1 head Savoy cabbage, leaves separated (scraps kept)
- 1 (23 oz) canned chopped tomatoes

Directions:

1. Melt the plant butter in a large bowl and cook the tofu until golden brown, 8 minutes. Stir in the onion and garlic until softened and fragrant, 3 minutes. Season with

salt, black pepper, and mix in the buckwheat, bay leaf, and vegetable stock.

2. Close the lid, allow boiling, and then simmer until all the liquid is absorbed. Open the lid; remove the bay leaf, adjust the taste with salt, black pepper, and mix in the cilantro.

3. Lay the cabbage leaves on a flat surface and add 3 to 4 tablespoons of the cooked buckwheat onto each leaf. Roll the leaves to firmly secure the filling.

4. Pour the tomatoes with juices into a medium pot, season with a little salt, black pepper, and lay the cabbage rolls in the sauce. Cook over medium heat until the cabbage softens, 5 to 8 minutes. Turn the heat off and dish the food onto serving plates. Garnish with more cilantro and serve warm.

Nutrition:

Calories 1147 | Fats 112. 9g | Carbs 25. 6g | Protein 23. 8g

Bbq Black Bean Burgers

Preparation Time: 15-30 minutes | Cooking Time: 20 minutes | Servings: 4

Ingredients:

- 3 (15 oz) cans black beans, drained and rinsed
- 2 tbsp whole-wheat flour
- 2 tbsp quick-cooking oats
- ¼ cup chopped fresh basil
- 2 tbsp pure barbecue sauce
- 1 garlic clove, minced
- Salt and black pepper to taste
- 4 whole-grain hamburger buns, split
- For topping:
- Red onion slices
- Tomato slices
- Fresh basil leaves
- Additional barbecue sauce

Directions:

1. In a medium bowl, mash the black beans and mix in the flour, oats, basil, barbecue sauce, garlic salt, and black

pepper until well combined. Mold 4 patties out of the mixture and set aside.

2. Heat a grill pan to medium heat and lightly grease with cooking spray.

3. Cook the bean patties on both sides until light brown and cooked through, 10 minutes.

4. Place the patties between the burger buns and top with the onions, tomatoes, basil, and some barbecue sauce.

5. Serve warm.

Nutrition:

Calories 589 | Fats 17. 7g | Carbs 80. 9g | Protein 27. 9g

Paprika & Tomato Pasta Primavera

Preparation Time: 15-30 minutes | Cooking Time: 25 minutes | Servings: 4

Ingredients:

- 2 tbsp olive oil
- 8 oz whole-wheat fedelini
- ½ tsp paprika
- 1 small red onion, sliced
- 2 garlic cloves, minced
- 1 cup dry white wine
- Salt and black pepper to taste
- 2 cups cherry tomatoes, halved
- 3 tbsp plant butter, cut into ½-in cubes
- 1 lemon, zested and juiced
- 1 cup packed fresh basil leaves

Directions:

1. Heat the olive oil in a large pot and mix in the fedelini, paprika, onion, garlic, and stir-fry for

2. 2-3 minutes.

3. Mix in the white wine, salt, and black pepper. Cover with water. Cook until the water absorbs

4. and the fedelini al dente, 5 minutes. Mix in the cherry tomatoes, plant butter, lemon zest,

5. lemon juice, and basil leaves.

6. Dish the food and serve warm.

Nutrition:

Calories 380 kcal |Fats 24. 1g | Carbs 33. 7g | Protein 11. 2g

Green Lentil Stew with Brown Rice

Preparation Time: 15-30 minutes | Cooking Time: 50 minutes | Servings: 4

Ingredients:

For the stew:

- 2 tbsp olive oil
- 1 lb tempeh, cut into cubes
- Salt and black pepper to taste
- 1 tsp chili powder
- 1 tsp onion powder
- 1 tsp cumin powder
- 1 tsp garlic powder
- 1 yellow onion, chopped
- 2 celery stalks, chopped
- 2 carrots diced
- 4 garlic cloves, minced
- 2 cups vegetable broth
- 1 tsp oregano
- 1 cup green lentils, rinsed
- ¼ cup chopped tomatoes
- 1 lime, juiced

For the brown rice:

- 1 cup of brown rice
- 1 cup of water
- Salt to taste

Directions:

- Heat the olive oil in a large pot, season the tempeh with salt, black pepper, and cook in the oil until brown, 10 minutes.
- Stir in the chili powder, onion powder, cumin powder, garlic powder, and cook until fragrant, 1 minute. Mix in the onion, celery, carrots, garlic, and cook until softened. Pour in the vegetable broth, oregano, green lentils, tomatoes, and green chilies.
- Cover the pot and cook until the tomatoes soften and the stew reduces by half, 10 to 15 minutes. Open the lid, adjust the taste with salt, black pepper, and mix in the lime juice. Dish the stew and serve warm with the brown rice.
- Meanwhile, as the stew cooks, add the brown rice, water, and salt to a medium pot. Cook over medium heat until the rice is tender and the water is absorbed for about 15 to 25 minutes.

Nutrition:

Calories 1305 kcal | Fats 130. 9g | Carbs 25. 1g | Protein 24. 3g

Dark Chocolate Quinoa Breakfast Bowl

Preparation Time: 15-30 minutes | Cooking Time: 30 minutes | Servings: 4

Ingredients:

- Uncooked white quinoa: 1 cup
- Unsweetened almond milk: 1 cup
- Coconut milk: 1 cup
- Sea salt: 1 pinch
- Unsweetened cocoa powder: 2 tbsp
- Maple syrup: 2-3 tbsp
- Pure vanilla extract: 1/2 tsp
- Vegan dark chocolate: 3-4 squares

Directions:

1. Rinse quinoa in a strainer
2. Heat the pan and add rinsed quinoa and dry them up
3. Add coconut milk, almond milk, and salt
4. Lower the heat to medium and stir gently for 20 minutes
5. Remove from heat after quinoa is tender

6. Add vanilla and maple syrup and serve

Nutrition:

Carbs: 40. 9 | Protein: 7. 5g | Fats: 6. 7g | Calories: 236 Kcal

Quinoa Black Beans Breakfast Bowl

Preparation Time: 5-15 minutes | Cooking Time: 25 minutes | Servings: 4

Ingredients:

- 1 cup brown quinoa, rinsed well
- Salt to taste
- 3 tbsp plant-based yogurt
- ½ lime, juiced
- 2 tbsp chopped fresh cilantro
- 1 (5 oz) can black beans, drained and rinsed
- 3 tbsp tomato salsa
- ¼ small avocado, pitted, peeled, and sliced
- 2 radishes, shredded
- 1 tbsp pepitas (pumpkin seeds)

Directions:

1. Cook the quinoa with 2 cups of slightly salted water in a medium pot over medium heat or until the liquid absorbs, 15 minutes.

2. Spoon the quinoa into serving bowls and fluff with a fork.
3. In a small bowl, mix the yogurt, lime juice, cilantro, and salt. Divide this mixture on the quinoa and top with the beans, salsa, avocado, radishes, and pepitas.
4. Serve immediately.

Nutrition:

Calories 131 | Fats 3. 5g | Carbs 20 | Protein 6. 5g

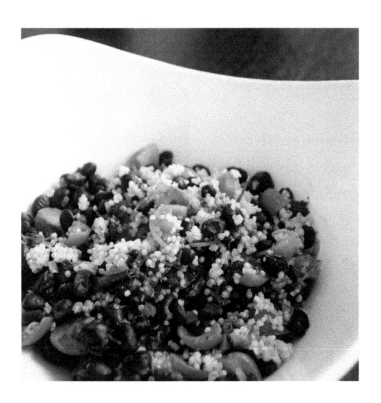

Corn Griddle Cakes With Tofu Mayonnaise

Preparation Time: 5-15 minutes | Cooking Time: 35 minutes | Servings: 4

Ingredients:

- 1 tbsp flax seed powder + 3 tbsp water
- 1 cup water or as needed
- 2 cups yellow cornmeal
- 1 tsp salt
- 2 tsp baking powder
- 4 tbsp olive oil for frying
- 1 cup tofu mayonnaise for serving

Directions:

1. In a medium bowl, mix the flax seed powder with water and allow thickening for 5 minutes to form the flax egg.
2. Mix in the water and then whisk in the cornmeal, salt, and baking powder until soup texture forms but not watery.

3. Heat a quarter of the olive oil in a griddle pan and pour in a quarter of the batter. Cook until set and golden brown beneath, 3 minutes. Flip the cake and cook the other side until set and golden brown too.
4. Plate the cake and make three more with the remaining oil and batter.
5. Top the cakes with some tofu mayonnaise before serving.

Nutrition:

Calories 896 | Fats 50. 7g | Carbs 91. 6g | Protein 17. 3g

Savory Breakfast Salad

Preparation Time: 15-30 minutes | Cooking Time: 20 minutes | Servings: 2

Ingredients:

- For the sweet potatoes:
- Sweet potato: 2 small
- Salt and pepper: 1 pinch
- Coconut oil: 1 tbsp
- For the Dressing:
- Lemon juice: 3 tbsp
- Salt and pepper: 1 pinch each
- Extra virgin olive oil: 1 tbsp
- For the Salad: Mixed greens: 4 cups
- For Servings: Hummus: 4 tbsp
- Blueberries: 1 cup
- Ripe avocado: 1 medium
- Fresh chopped parsley
- Hemp seeds: 2 tbsp

Directions:

1. Take a large skillet and apply gentle heat

2. Add sweet potatoes, coat them with salt and pepper and pour some oil
3. Cook till sweet potatoes turns browns
4. Take a bowl and mix lemon juice, salt, and pepper
5. Add salad, sweet potatoes, and the serving together
6. Mix well and dress and serve

Nutrition:

Carbs: 57. 6g | Protein: 7. 5g | Fats: 37. 6g | Calories: 523 Kcal

Almond Plum Oats Overnight

Preparation Time: 15-30 minutes | Cooking Time: 10 minutes plus overnight | Servings: 2

Ingredients:

- Rolled oats: 60g
- Plums: 3 ripe and chopped
- Almond milk: 300ml
- Chia seeds: 1 tbsp
- Nutmeg: a pinch
- Vanilla extract: a few drops
- Whole almonds: 1 tbsp roughly chopped

Directions:

1. Add oats, nutmeg, vanilla extract, almond milk, and chia seeds to a bowl and mix well • Add in cubed plums and cover and place in the fridge for a night
2. Mix the oats well next morning and add into the serving bowl
3. Serve with your favorite toppings

Nutrition:

Carbs: 24. 7g | Protein: 9. 5g | Fats: 10. 8g | Calories: 248Kcal

High Protein Toast

Preparation Time: 15-30 minutes | Cooking Time: 15 minutes |
Servings: 2

Ingredients:

- White bean: 1 drained and rinsed
- Cashew cream: ½ cup
- Miso paste: 1 ½ tbsp
- Toasted sesame oil: 1 tsp
- Sesame seeds: 1 tbsp
- Spring onion: 1 finely sliced
- Lemon: 1 half for the juice and half wedged to serve
- Rye bread: 4 slices toasted

Directions:

1. In a bowl add sesame oil, white beans, miso, cashew cream, and lemon juice and mash using a potato masher
2. Make a spread
3. Spread it on a toast and top with spring onions and sesame seeds
4. Serve with lemon wedges

Nutrition:

Carbs: 44. 05 g | Protein: 14. 05 g | Fats: 9. 25 g | Calories: 332 Kcal

Hummus Carrot Sandwich

Preparation Time: 15-30 minutes | Cooking Time: 25 minutes | Servings: 2

Ingredients:

- Chickpeas: 1 cup can drain and rinsed
- Tomato: 1 small sliced
- Cucumber: 1 sliced
- Avocado: 1 sliced
- Cumin: 1 tsp
- Carrot: 1 cup diced
- Maple syrup: 1 tsp
- Tahini: 3 tbsp
- Garlic: 1 clove
- Lemon: 2 tbsp
- Extra-virgin olive oil: 2 tbsp
- Salt: as per your need
- Bread slices: 4

Directions:

1. Add carrot to the boiling hot water and boil for 15 minutes

2. Blend boiled carrots, maple syrup, cumin, chickpeas, tahini, olive oil, salt, and garlic together

3. in a blender

4. Add in lemon juice and mix

5. Add to the serving bowl and you can refrigerate for up to 5 days

6. In between two bread slices, spread hummus and place 2-3 slices of cucumber, avocado, and

7. tomato and serve

Nutrition:

Carbs: 53. 15 g | Protein: 14. 1 g | Fats: 27. 5 g | Calories: 490 Kcal

Overnight Oats

Preparation Time: 15-30 minutes | Cooking Time: 15 minutes plus overnight | Servings: 6

Ingredients:

- Cinnamon: a pinch
- Almond milk: 600ml
- Porridge oats: 320g Maple syrup: 1 tbsp
- Pumpkin seeds 1 tbsp
- Chia seeds: 1 tbsp

Directions:

1. Add all the ingredients to the bowl and combine well
2. Cover the bowl and place it in the fridge overnight
3. Pour more milk in the morning Serve with your favorite toppings

Nutrition:

Carbs: 32. 3 g | Protein: 10. 2 g | Fats: 12. 7 g | Calories: 298 Kcal

Avocado Miso Chickpeas Toast

Preparation Time: 15-30 minutes | Cooking Time: 15 minutes |
Servings: 2

Ingredients:

- Chickpeas: 400g drained and rinsed
- Avocado: 1 medium
- Toasted sesame oil: 1 tsp
- White miso paste: 1 ½ tbsp
- Sesame seeds: 1 tbsp
- Spring onion: 1 finely sliced
- Lemon: 1 half for the juice and half wedged to serve
- Rye bread: 4 slices toasted

Directions:

1. In a bowl add sesame oil, chickpeas, miso, and lemon juice and mash using a potato masher • Roughly crushed avocado in another bowl using a fork
2. Add the avocado to the chickpeas and make a spread
3. Spread it on a toast and top with spring onion and sesame seeds
4. Serve with lemon wedges

Nutrition:

Carbs: 33. 3 g | Protein: 14. 6 g | Fats: 26. 6 g | Calories: 456 Kcal

Banana Malt Bread

Preparation Time: 15-30 minutes | Cooking Time: 1 hour 20 minutes and Maturing Time | Servings: 12 slices

Ingredients:

- Hot strong black tea: 120ml
- Malt extract: 150g plus extra for brushing Bananas: 2 ripe mashed
- Sultanas: 100g Pitted dates: 120g chopped
- Plain flour: 250g Soft dark brown sugar: 50g Baking powder: 2 tsp

Directions:

1. Preheat the oven to 140C
2. Line the loaf tin with the baking paper
3. Brew tea and include sultanas and dates to it
4. Take a small pan and heat the malt extract and gradually add sugar to it
5. Stir continuously and let it cook
6. In a bowl, add flour, salt, and baking powder and now top with sugar extract, fruits, bananas,
7. and tea

8. Mix the batter well and add to the loaf tin

9. Bake the mixture for an hour

10. Brush the bread with extra malt extract and let it cool down before removing from the tin • When done, wrap in a foil; it can be consumed for a week

Nutrition:

Carbs: 43. 3 g | Protein: 3. 4 g | Fats: 0. 3 g | Calories: 194 Kcal

Banana Vegan Bread

Preparation Time: 15-30 minutes | Cooking Time: 1 hour 15 minutes | Servings: 1 loaf

Ingredients:

- Overripe banana:
- 3 large mashed
- All-purpose flour: 200 g Unsweetened non-dairy milk: 50 ml
- White vinegar: ½ tsp
- Ground flaxseed: 10 g Ground cinnamon: ¼ tsp
- Granulated sugar: 140 g Vanilla: ¼ tsp
- Baking powder: ¼ tsp
- Baking soda: ¼ tsp
- Salt: ¼ tsp
- Canola oil: 3 tbsp
- Chopped walnuts: ½ cup

Directions:

1. Preheat the oven to 350F and line the loaf pan with parchment paper
2. Mash bananas using a fork

3. Take a large bowl, and add in mash bananas, canola oil, oat milk, sugar, vinegar, vanilla, and
4. ground flax seed
5. Also whisk in baking powder, cinnamon, flour, and salt
6. Add batter to the loaf pan and bake for 50 minutes
7. Remove from pan and let it sit for 10 minutes
8. Slice when completely cooled down

Nutrition:

Carbs: 40. 3g | Protein: 2. 8g | Fats: 8. 2g | Calories: 240Kcal

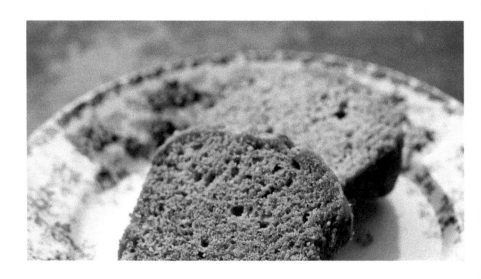

Berry Compote Pancakes

Preparation Time: 15-30 minutes | Cooking Time: 30 minutes | Servings: 2

Ingredients:

- Mixed frozen berries: 200g
- Plain flour: 140 g
- Unsweetened almond milk: 140ml
- Icing sugar: 1 tbsp
- Lemon juice: 1 tbsp
- Baking powder: 2 tsp
- Vanilla extract: a dash
- Salt: a pinch
- Caster sugar: 2 tbsp
- Vegetable oil: ½ tbsp

Directions:

1. Take a small pan and add berries, lemon juice, and icing sugar
2. Cook the mixture for 10 minutes to give it a saucy texture and set aside

3. Take a bowl and add caster sugar, flour, baking powder, and salt and mix well
4. Add in almond milk and vanilla and combine well to make a batter
5. Take a non-stick pan, and heat 2 teaspoons oil in it and spread it over the whole surface
6. Add ¼ cup of the batter to the pan and cook each side for 3-4 minutes
7. Serve with compote

Nutrition:

Carbs: 92 g | Protein: 9. 4 g | Fats: 5. 2 g | Calories: 463 Kcal

Southwest Breakfast Bowl

Preparation Time: 15-30 minutes | Cooking Time: 15 minutes | Servings: 1

Ingredients:

- Mushrooms: 1 cup sliced
- Chopped cilantro: ½ cup
- Chili powder: 1 tsp
- Red pepper: 1/2 diced
- Zucchini: 1 cup diced
- Green onion: 1/2 cup chopped
- Onion: 1/2 cup
- Vegan sausage: 1 sliced
- Garlic powder: 1 tsp
- Paprika: 1 tsp
- Cumin: 1/2 tsp
- Salt and pepper: as per your taste
- Avocado: for topping

Directions:

1. Put everything in a bowl and apply gentle heat until vegetables turn brown

2. Pour some pepper and salt as you like and serve with your favorite toppings

Nutrition:

Carbs: 31. 6g | Protein: 33. 8g | Fats: 12. 2g | Calories: 361

Buckwheat Crepes

Preparation Time: 15-30 minutes | Cooking Time: 25 minutes | Servings: 12

Ingredients:

- Raw buckwheat flour: 1 cup
- Light coconut milk: 1 and 3/4 cups
- Ground cinnamon: 1/8 tsp
- Flaxseeds: 3/4 tbsp
- Melted coconut oil: 1 tbsp
- Sea salt: a pinch
- Any sweetener: as per your taste

Directions:

1. Take a bowl and add flaxseed, coconut milk, salt, avocado, and cinnamon Mix them all well and fold in the flour
2. Now take a nonstick pan and pour oil and provide gentle heat
3. Add a big spoon of a mixture
4. Cook till it appears bubbly, then change side
5. Perform the task until all crepes are prepared
6. For enhancing the taste, add the sweetener of your liking

Nutrition:

Carbs: 8g | Protein: 1g | Fats: 3g | Calories: 71Kcal

Chickpeas Spread Sourdough Toast

Preparation Time: 15-30 minutes | Cooking Time: 15 minutes | Servings: 4

Ingredients:

- Chickpeas: 1 cup rinsed and drained
- Pumpkin puree: 1 cup
- Vegan yogurt: ½ cup
- Salt: as per your need
- Sourdough: 4 slices toasted

Directions:

1. In a bowl add chickpeas and pumpkin puree and mash using a potato masher
2. Add in salt and yogurt and mix
3. Spread it on a toast and serve

Nutrition:

Carbs: 33. 7g | Protein: 8. 45g | Fats: 2. 5g | Calories: 187Kcal

Chickpeas with Harissa

Preparation Time: 15-30 minutes | Cooking Time: 20 minutes | Servings: 2

Ingredients:

- Chickpeas: 1 cup can rinse and drained well
- Onion: 1 small diced
- Cucumber: 1 cup diced
- Tomato: 1 cup diced
- Salt: as per your taste
- Lemon juice: 2 tbsp
- Harissa: 2 tsp
- Olive oil: 1 tbsp
- Flat-leaf parsley: 2 tbsp chopped

Directions:

1. Add lemon juice, harissa, and olive oil in a bowl and whisk
2. Take a serving bowl and add onion, cucumber, chickpeas, salt and the sauce you made
3. Add parsley from the top and serve

Nutrition:

Carbs: 55. 6 g | Protein: 17. 8g | Fats: 11. 8g | Calories: 398Kcal

Chocolate Chip Pancake

Preparation Time: 15-30 minutes | Cooking Time: 30 minutes | Servings: 6 pancakes

Ingredients:

- All-purpose flour: 140g
- Melted coconut oil: 1 tbsp
- Vegan sugar: 2 tbsp
- Warm almond milk: 250ml
- Baking powder: 1 tbsp
- Sea salt: ¼ tsp
- Chocolate chips: 2 tbsp

Directions:

1. Combine together flour, salt, and baking powder and add in chocolate chips
2. Warm almond milk in the microwave and add sugar and coconut oil and mix well
3. There should be no lump in the batter
4. Combine together now dry ingredients and the wet ingredients
5. Add oil to the non-stick pan on medium heat

6. Add ¼ cup of the batter to the pan and cook each side for 3-4 minutes
7. Serve with vegan butter or any topping you like

Nutrition:

Amount Per 1 Pancake

Carbs: 29. 4 g | Protein: 3. 1 g | Fats: 5 g | Calories: 167 Kcal

Coconut, Raspberry, and Chocolate Porridge

Preparation Time: 15-30 minutes | Cooking Time: 20 minutes | Servings: 2

Ingredients:

- Almond milk: 300 ml
- Quinoa: 80 g
- Coconut water: 100ml
- Raspberries: 100g
- Cocoa powder: 1 tbsp
- Coconut sugar: 2 tbsp
- Cocoa nibs: 2 tbsp
- Vegan coconut chips: 2 tbsp toasted

Directions:

1. Take a small pan and add coconut water, quinoa, coconut sugar, almond milk, and cocoa powder
2. Heat the pan for 20 minutes over medium heat
3. Stir continuously in between

4. Top with cocoa nibs, coconut chips, and raspberries and serve

Nutrition:

Carbs: 45. 3 g | Protein: 10. 3 g | Fats: 19. 3 g | Calories: 415 Kcal

Toasted Rye with Pumpkin Seed Butter

Preparation Time: 15-30 minutes | Cooking Time: 25 minutes and the cooling time | Servings: 4

Ingredients:

- Pumpkin seeds: 220g
- Date nectar: 1 tsp
- Avocado oil: 2 tbsp
- Rye bread: 4 slices toasted

Directions:

1. Toast the pumpkin seed on a frying pan on low heat for 5-7 minutes and stir in between
2. Let them turn golden and remove from pan
3. Add to the blender, when they cool down and make fine powder
4. Add in avocado oil and salt and then again blend to form a paste
5. Add date nectars too and blend
6. On the toasted rye, spread one tablespoon of this butter and serve with your favorite toppings

Nutrition:

Carbs: 3 g | Protein: 5 g | Fats: 10. 3 g | Calories: 127 Kcal

Vegan Breakfast Hash

Preparation Time: 15-30 minutes | Cooking Time: 25 minutes | Servings: 4

Ingredients:

- Bell Pepper: 1
- Smoked Paprika: ½ tsp
- Potatoes: 3 medium
- Mushrooms: 8 oz
- Yellow Onion: 1
- Zucchini: 1
- Cumin Powder: ½ tsp
- Garlic Powder: ½ tsp
- Salt and Pepper: as per your taste
- Cooking oil: 2 tbsp (optional)

Directions:

1. Heat a large pan on medium flame, add oil and put the sliced potatoes
2. Cook the potatoes till they change color
3. Cut the rest of the vegetables and add all the spices
4. Cooked till veggies are soften

Nutrition:

Carbs: 29. 7g | Protein: 5. 5g | Fats: 10g | Calories: 217 Kcal

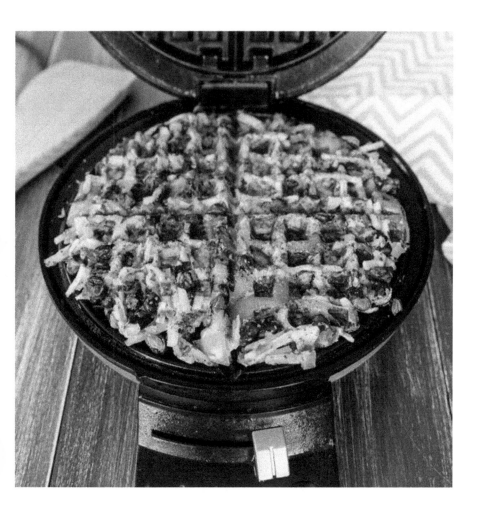

Vegan Muffins Breakfast Sandwich

Preparation Time: 15-30 minutes | Cooking Time: 20 minutes | Servings: 2

Ingredients:

- Romesco Sauce: 3-4 tablespoons
- Fresh baby spinach: ½ cup
- Tofu Scramble: 2
- Vegan English muffins: 2
- Avocado: ½ peeled and sliced
- Sliced fresh tomato: 1

Directions:

1. In the oven, toast English muffin
2. Half the muffin and spread romesco sauce
3. Paste spinach to one side, tailed by avocado slices
4. Have warm tofu followed by a tomato slice
5. Place the other muffin half onto to the preceding one

Nutrition:

Carbs: 18g | Protein: 12g | Fats: 14g | Calories: 276 Kcal

Almond Waffles With Cranberries

Preparation Time: 5-15 minutes | Cooking Time: 20 minutes | Servings: 4

Ingredients:

- 2 tbsp flax seed powder + 6 tbsp water
- 2/3 cup almond flour
- 2 ½ tsp baking powder
- A pinch salt
- 1 ½ cups almond milk
- 2 tbsp plant butter
- 1 cup fresh almond butter
- 2 tbsp pure maple syrup
- 1 tsp fresh lemon juice

Directions:

1. In a medium bowl, mix the flax seed powder with water and allow soaking for 5 minutes.
2. Add the almond flour, baking powder, salt, and almond milk.

3. Mix until well combined.
4. Preheat a waffle iron and brush with some plant butter.
5. Pour in a quarter cup of the batter,
6. close the iron and cook until the waffles are golden and crisp, 2 to 3 minutes.
7. Transfer the waffles to a plate and make more waffles using the same process and ingredient
8. proportions.
9. Meanwhile, in a medium bowl, mix the almond butter with the maple syrup and lemon juice.
10. Serve the waffles, spread the top with the almond-lemon mixture, and serve.

Nutrition:

Calories 533 | Fats 53g | Carbs 16. 7g | Protein 1. 2g

Chickpea Omelet with Spinach and Mushrooms

Preparation Time: 5-15 minutes | Cooking Time: 25 minutes | Servings: 4

Ingredients:

- 1 cup chickpea flour
- ½ tsp onion powder
- ½ tsp garlic powder
- ¼ tsp white pepper
- ¼ tsp black pepper
- 1/3 cup nutritional yeast
- ½ tsp baking soda
- 1 small green bell pepper, deseeded and chopped
- 3 scallions, chopped
- 1 cup sautéed sliced white button mushrooms
- ½ cup chopped fresh spinach
- 1 cup halved cherry tomatoes for serving
- 1 tbsp fresh parsley leaves

Directions:

1. In a medium bowl, mix the chickpea flour, onion powder, garlic powder, white pepper, black pepper, nutritional yeast, and baking soda until well combined.
2. Heat a medium skillet over medium heat and add a quarter of the batter.
3. Swirl the pan to spread the batter across the pan.
4. Scatter a quarter each of the bell pepper, scallions, mushrooms, and spinach on top, and cook until the bottom part of the omelet sets and is golden brown, 1 to 2 minutes.
5. Carefully, flip the omelet and cook the other side until set and golden brown.
6. Transfer the omelet to a plate and make the remaining omelets using the remaining batter in the same proportions.
7. Serve the omelet with the tomatoes and garnish with the parsley leaves. Serve.

Nutrition:

Calories 147 | Fats 1. 8g | Carbs 21. 3g | Protein 11. 6g

Sweet Coconut Raspberry Pancakes

Preparation Time: 5-15 minutes | Cooking Time: 25 minutes | Servings: 4

Ingredients:

- 2 tbsp flax seed powder + 6 tbsp water
- ½ cup of coconut milk
- ¼ cup fresh raspberries, mashed
- ½ cup oat flour
- 1 tsp baking soda
- A pinch salt
- 1 tbsp coconut sugar
- 2 tbsp pure date syrup
- ½ tsp cinnamon powder
- 2 tbsp unsweetened coconut flakes
- 2 tsp plant butter
- Fresh raspberries for garnishing

Directions:

1. In a medium bowl, mix the flax seed powder with the water and allow thickening for 5 minutes.
2. Mix in the coconut milk and raspberries.
3. Add the oat flour, baking soda, salt, coconut sugar, date syrup, and cinnamon powder.
4. Fold in the coconut flakes until well combined.
5. Working in batches, melt a quarter of the butter in a non-stick skillet and add ¼ cup of the batter.
6. Cook until set beneath and golden brown, 2 minutes.
7. Flip the pancake and cook on the other side until set and golden brown, 2 minutes.
8. Transfer to a plate and make the remaining pancakes using the rest of the ingredients in the same proportions.
9. Garnish the pancakes with some raspberries and serve warm!

Nutrition:

Calories 412 | Fats 28. 3g | Carbs 33. 7g | Protein 7. 6g

Pumpkin-Pistachio Tea Cake

Preparation Time: 5-15 minutes | Cooking Time: 70 minutes | Servings: 4

Ingredients:

- 2 tbsp flaxseed powder + 6 tbsp water
- 3 tbsp vegetable oil
- ¾ cup canned unsweetened pumpkin puree
- ½ cup pure corn syrup
- 3 tbsp pure date sugar
- 1 ½ cups whole-wheat flour
- ½ tsp cinnamon powder
- ½ tsp baking powder
- ¼ tsp cloves powder
- ½ tsp allspice powder
- ½ tsp nutmeg powder
- A pinch salt
- 2 tbsp chopped pistachios

Directions:

1. Preheat the oven to 350 F and lightly coat an 8 x 4-inch loaf pan with cooking spray.

2. In a medium bowl, mix the flax seed powder with water and allow thickening for 5 minutes to make the flax egg.

3. In a bowl, whisk the vegetable oil, pumpkin puree, corn syrup, date sugar, and flax egg.

4. In another bowl, mix the flour, cinnamon powder, baking powder, cloves powder, allspice powder, nutmeg powder, and salt.

5. Add this mixture to the wet batter and mix until well combined.

6. Pour the batter into the loaf pan, sprinkle the pistachios on top, and gently press the nuts onto the batter to stick.

7. Bake in the oven for 50 to 55 minutes or until a toothpick inserted into the cake comes out clean.

8. Remove the cake onto a wire rack, allow cooling, slice, and serve.

Nutrition:

Calories 330 | Fats 13. 2g | Carbs 50. 1g | Protein 7g

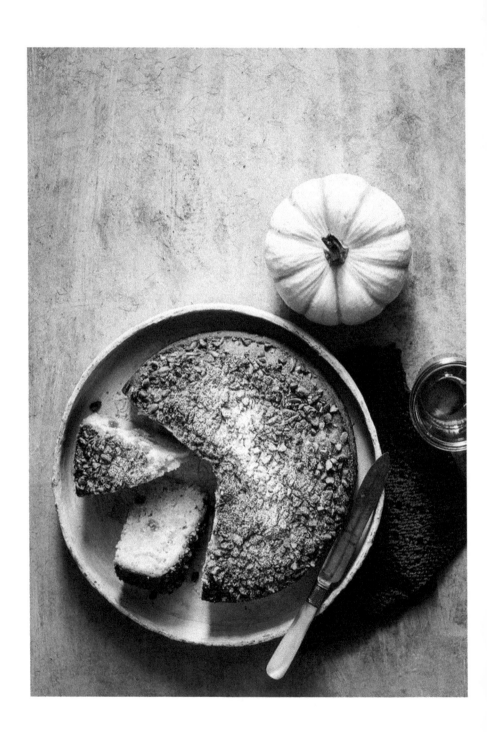

Lightning Source UK Ltd.
Milton Keynes UK
UKHW020811110621
385331UK00004B/119